The Inspired Plant-Based Lunch Cookbook

Fit and Tasty Lunch Recipes to Start Your Plant-Based Diet and Improve Your Health

Carl Brady

Table of contents

Cabbage Stew

Preparation time: 10 minutes Cooking time: 50 minutes
Servings: 6

Ingredients:

12 ounces cooked Cannellini beans 8 ounces smoked tofu, firm, sliced 1 medium cabbage, chopped 1 large white onion, peeled, julienned 2 ½ teaspoon minced garlic 1 tablespoon sweet paprika 5 tablespoons tomato paste 3 teaspoons smoked paprika 1/3 teaspoon ground black pepper 2 teaspoons dried thyme 2/3 teaspoon salt ½ tsp ground coriander 3 bay leaves 4 tablespoons olive oil 1 cup vegetable broth

Directions:

Take a large saucepan, place it over medium heat, add 3 tablespoons oil and when hot, add onion and garlic and cook for 3 minutes or until saute. Add cabbage, pour in water, simmer for 10 minutes or until softened, then stir in all the spices and continue cooking for 30 minutes. Add beans and tomato paste, pour in water, stir until mixed and cook for 15 minutes until thoroughly cooked. Take a separate skillet pan, add 1 tablespoon oil and when hot, add tofu slices and cook for 5 minutes until golden brown on both sides. Serve cooked cabbage stew with fried tofu.

African Peanut Lentil Soup

Preparation time: 10 minutes Cooking time: 25 minutes
Servings: 3

Ingredients:

1/2 cup red lentils

1/2 medium white onion, sliced

2 medium tomatoes, chopped

1/2 cup baby spinach

1/2 cup sliced zucchini

1/2 cup sliced sweet potatoes

½ cup sliced potatoes

½ cup broccoli florets

2 teaspoons minced garlic

1 inch of ginger, grated

1 tablespoon tomato paste

1/4 teaspoon ground black pepper

1 teaspoon salt

1 ½ teaspoon ground cumin

2 teaspoons ground coriander

2 tablespoons peanuts 1 teaspoon Harissa Spice Blend

1 tablespoon sambal oelek

1/4 cup almond butter

1 teaspoon olive oil

1 teaspoon lemon juice

2 ½ cups vegetable stock

Directions:

Take a large saucepan, place it over medium heat, add oil and when hot, add onion and cook for 5 minutes until translucent. Meanwhile, place tomatoes in a blender, add garlic, ginger and sambal oelek along with all the spices and pulse until pureed. Pour this mixture into the onions, cook for 5 minutes, then add remaining ingredients except for spinach, peanuts and lemon juice and simmer for 15 minutes. Taste to adjust the seasoning, stir in spinach, and cook for 5 minutes until cooked. Ladle soup into bowls, garnish with lime juice and peanuts and serve

Eggplant, Onion and Tomato Stew

Preparation time: 5 minutes Cooking time: 5 minutes Servings: 4

Ingredients:

3 1/2 cups cubed eggplant 1 cup diced white onion 2 cups diced tomatoes 1 teaspoon ground cumin 1/8 teaspoon ground cayenne pepper 1 teaspoon salt 1 cup tomato sauce 1/2 cup water

Directions:

Switch on the instant pot, place all the ingredients in it, stir until mixed, and seal the pot. Press the 'manual' button and cook for 5 minutes at high-pressure setting until cooked. When done, do quick pressure release, open the instant pot, and stir the stew. Serve straight away.

Brussel Sprouts Stew

Preparation time: 10 minutes Cooking time: 55 minutes Servings: 4

Ingredients:

35 ounces Brussels sprouts 5 medium potato, peeled, chopped 1 medium onion, peeled, chopped 2 carrot, peeled, cubed 2 teaspoon smoked paprika 1/8 teaspoon ground black pepper 1/8 teaspoon salt 3 tablespoons caraway seeds 1/2 teaspoon red chili powder 1 tablespoon nutmeg 1 tablespoon olive oil 4 ½ cups hot vegetable stock

Directions:

Take a large pot, place it over medium-high heat, add oil and when hot, add onion and cook for 1 minute. Then add carrot and potato, cook for 2 minutes, then add Brussel sprouts and cook for 5 minutes. Stir in all the spices, pour in vegetable stock, bring the mixture to boil, switch heat to medium-low and simmer for 45 minutes until cooked and stew reach to desired thickness. Serve straight away.

Black Bean and Quinoa Stew

Preparation time: 10 minutes Cooking time: 6 hours Servings: 6

Ingredients:

1 pound black beans, dried, soaked overnight 3/4 cup quinoa, uncooked 1 medium red bell pepper, cored, chopped 1 medium red onion, peeled, diced 1 medium green bell pepper, cored, chopped 28-ounce diced tomatoes 2 dried chipotle peppers 1 ½ teaspoon minced garlic 2/3 teaspoon sea salt 2 teaspoons red chili powder 1/3 teaspoon ground black pepper 1 teaspoon coriander powder 1 dried cinnamon stick 1/4 cup cilantro 7 cups of water

Directions: Switch on the slow cooker, add all the ingredients in it, except for salt, and stir until mixed. Shut the cooker with lid and cook for 6 hours at a high heat setting until cooked. When done, stir salt into the stew until mixed, remove cinnamon sticks and serve

Portobello Mushroom Stew

Preparation time: 10 minutes Cooking time: 8 hours Servings: 4

Ingredients:

8 cups vegetable broth 1 cup dried wild mushrooms 1 cup dried chickpeas 3 cups chopped potato 2 cups chopped carrots 1 cup corn kernels 2 cups diced white onions 1 tablespoon minced parsley 3 cups chopped zucchini 1 tablespoon minced rosemary 1 1/2 teaspoon ground black pepper 1 teaspoon dried sage 2/3 teaspoon salt 1 teaspoon dried oregano 3 tablespoons soy sauce 1 1/2 teaspoons liquid smoke 8 ounces tomato paste

Directions: Switch on the slow cooker, add all the ingredients in it, and stir until mixed. Shut the cooker with lid and cook for 10 hours at a high heat setting until cooked. Serve straight away. Nutrition Value: Calories: 447 Cal Fat: 36 g Carbs: 24 g Protein: 11 g Fiber: 2 g

Greens Salad with Black Eyed Peas

Preparation time: 5 minutes Cooking time: 6 minutes Servings: 3

Ingredients:

2 cups cooked black-eyed peas, cooked 1/2 cup cooked quinoa 3 cups chopped purple cabbage 5 cups chopped kale 1/2 of a shallot, peeled, chopped 1 1/2 cup shredded carrot 1 teaspoon minced garlic 1/2 teaspoon sea salt 1/3 teaspoon ground black pepper 1 tablespoon apple cider vinegar and more as needed 1 tablespoon lemon juice 2 tablespoons olive oil

Directions:

Sauté garlic, shallot, and cabbage in 1 tablespoon for 2 minutes over medium heat, then add remaining oil along with kale, season with salt, and cook for 4 minutes until kale has wilted. Transfer the vegetables to a bowl, add remaining ingredients and toss until combined. Serve straight away.

Moo Goo Gai Pan

Preparation time: 10 minutes Cooking time: 40 minutes
Servings: 4

Ingredients:

Marinade: 2 Tablespoons Soy Sauce, Lite 2 Tablespoons Vegetable Stock 1 Tablespoon Sesame Oil 1 Clove Garlic, Minced ½ Inch Ginger, Fresh, Peeled & Grated

Stir Fry: 14 Ounces Firm Tofu, Pressed Overnight & Cubed 1 Tablespoon Sesame Oil 8 Ounces White Mushrooms, Sliced 1 Carrot, Julienned 1 Cup Sugar Snap Peas, Rinsed & Trimmed 1 Clove Garlic, Minced 1 Cup Vegetable Stock 1 Inch Piece Ginger, Peeled & Grated 2 Tablespoons Soy Sauce 8 Ounces Water Chestnuts, Canned, Sliced & Drained 8 Ounces Bamboo Shoots, Canned & Drained 1 Tablespoon Cornstarch 1/3 Cup Hot Water Cooked Noodles for Serving

Directions:

Start by making your marinade by whisking all ingredients together, and then add in your tofu. Allow it to marinate for thirty minutes. Press sauté and set it to low, and then add in the oil. Once it's hot add in the marinated tofu, and cook for ten minutes. Remove your tofu and place it to the side. Turn your instant pot off of sauté and then add in your carrot, garlic, ginger, snap peas, mushrooms, stock, soy sauce, bamboo shoots and water chestnuts. Stir well. Press sauté and select low once more, and cover your pot using a tempered glass lid, letting it simmer for five minutes. Stir often. Get out a bowl and whisk the water and cornstarch together to make a slurry. Add it to the pot, and then simmer while uncovered for five minutes Serve over noodles.

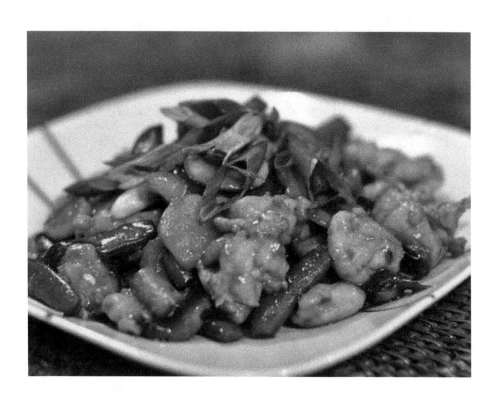

Cauliflower Red Curry

Preparation time: 10 minutes Cooking time: 30 minutes
Servings: 4

Ingredients:

2 Tablespoons Red Curry Paste 1 Teaspoon Garlic Powder 1 Cup Water 14 Ounces Coconut Milk, Canned & Full Fat Sea Salt & Black Pepper to Taste ¼ Teaspoon Chili Powder ½ Teaspoon Ginger 1 Bell Pepper, Sliced Thin 1 Cauliflower Head, Chopped 14 Ounces Tomatoes with Liquid, Canned & Diced Cooked Rice for Serving

Directions:

Stir your red curry paste, garlic powder, salt, ginger, onion powder chili powder, water, and coconut milk together in your instant pot. Throw in your cauliflower, tomatoes and bell pepper next. Stir well, and then seal the lid. Cook on high pressure for two minutes. Use a quick release, and stir well before serving over rice.

Lasagna Soup

Preparation time: 10 minutes Cooking time: 40 minutes Servings: 4

Ingredients:

2 Tablespoons Olive Oil

1 Onion, Diced

1 Clove Garlic, Diced

2 Teaspoons Oregano

1 Teaspoon Rosemary

¾ Teaspoons Red Pepper Flakes

½ Teaspoon Sea Salt, Fine

2 Tomatoes, Chopped

1 Cube Vegetable Bouillon

1 Bay Leaf 10 Lasagna Noodles, Broken

2/3 Cup Red Sauce

6 Cups Water Sea Salt & Black Pepper to Taste

Basil, Fresh for Garnish Shredded

Vegan Cheese for Garnish

Directions:

Press sauté, and then add in the oil. Heat until it begins to shimmer, and then throw in your onion. Cook for three minutes before tossing in your garlic. Cook for another minute, and stir often to keep it from burning. Add the rosemary, red pepper flakes, oregano, salt, bouillon cube, tomatoes, bay leaf, noodles, water and red sauce. Stir well, and make sure that your noodles are completely submerged. Seal the lid, and then cook on high pressure for four minutes. Use a natural pressure release for ten minutes before finishing with a quick release. Discard the bay leaf, and season with salt and pepper before serving garnished with basil and vegan cheese.

26

Apple Cider Vinegar Main:

8 Ounces Stir Fry Noodles 2 Cups Pea Pods, Fresh 4 Carrots, Julienned 2 Red Peppers, Sliced ½ Red Onion, Sliced Toppings: Cilantro Peanuts Lime Juice

Directions:

Start by combining all of your sauce ingredients in your instant pot and then press sauté. Once it starts to boil, stir the noodles in. allow it to simmer for three minutes, but make sure to stir often. Turn the instant pot off of sauté. Then seal the lid, and cook on high pressure for a minute. Use a quick release, and then combine your vegetables. Mix well and garnish before serving warm.

Beets, Edamame & Mixed Green Salad

Preparation Time: 10 minutes Cooking Time: 0 minute
Serving: 1

Ingredients:

2 cups mixed greens ½ raw beet, peeled and shredded 1 cup shelled edamame, thawed 1 tablespoon red wine vinegar 1 tablespoon fresh cilantro, chopped 2 teaspoons extra-virgin olive oil Pepper to taste

Directions:

Place the mixed greens in a food container. Top with shredded beets and edamame. In a glass jar with lid, mix the rest of the Ingredients. Refrigerate the salad and drizzle with the dressing when ready to eat.

Black Bean & Corn Salad

Preparation Time: 15 minutes Cooking Time: 0 minute Servings: 4

Ingredients:

2 tablespoons olive oil ¼ cup lime juice ¼ cup fresh cilantro, chopped Salt and pepper to taste 2 cups red cabbage, shredded 2 ¼ cups corn kernels ⅓ cup pine nuts, toasted 30 oz. canned black beans, rinsed and drained 1 tomato, diced ½ cup red onion, minced

Directions:

In a glass jar with lid, blend the oil, lime juice, cilantro, salt and pepper. In a food container, arrange the red cabbage, topped with the rest of the Ingredients. Cover and refrigerate until ready to serve. Drizzle with dressing before serving.

Cheese Paste

Preparation Time: 30minutes

Ingredients:

1/2 cup chopped red peppers 2 tbsp water 2 tbsp Nutritional yeast 2 tbsp freshly squeezed lemon juice 3/4 teaspoon Himalayan crystal salt or sea salt 1/4 tsp paprika powder 1/4 teaspoon smoked paprika powder 1/4 teaspoon turmeric powder 2 large pinches of cayenne 1 cup finely ground cashews

Directions:

Combine red peppers, water, yeast, lemon juice, salt, paprika powder, smoked paprika, turmeric powder, cayenne pepper and finely ground cashews in a blender. Mix until smooth.

Zucchini Balsamic Vinegar Burgers

Preparation time: 10 minutes Cooking time: 50 minutes
Servings 4–6 burgers

Ingredients:

1 zucchini, cut in 1/4 inch thick slices 2 tablespoons olive oil 1 tablespoon balsamic vinegar Salt, pepper

Directions: To take the bitterness out of zucchini, there is a simple process. Place the zucchini slices in a colander and sprinkle slices with an ample amount of salt. Leave the zucchini with salt in colander for thirty minutes. Rinse the zucchini and dab them dry with paper towels. Place in mixing bowl, drizzle olive oil over slices and toss until evenly coated. Add one tablespoon of olive oil to frying pan and heat over medium. Cook burgers on each side 4 minutes, until golden in color. Remove from heat and soak in balsamic vinegar, salt and pepper. Serve delicious slices over your favorite choice of bread and toppings.

Tofu Portobello Burgers

Preparation time: 10 minutes Cooking time: 60 minutes

Servings 4 burgers

Ingredients:

4 Portobello mushrooms 1 large red onion, sliced 1 tablespoon balsamic vinegar 2 garlic cloves, minced 2 tablespoons olive oil 10 oz firm packed tofu 1/2 cup red wine 1 tablespoon soy sauce 1 teaspoon agave syrup 1 tablespoon sesame seeds

Directions: In a medium mixing bowl, whisk together the four ingredients below the tofu in the list, include a dash of freshly ground pepper. Slice the tofu and place in mixture for thirty minutes to infuse with flavor. Prepare the portabellas for cooking by slicing and removing stems. Fry the mushrooms over medium heat until cooked through. Remove mushrooms and place tofu in same pan. Cook until browned. Mix together the remaining ingredients. Layer ingredients and marinade over bread and serve.

Chickpeas Burgers

Preparation time:

10 minutes Cooking time: 40 minutes Servings 6–8 burgers

Ingredients:

3 oz bulgur 2 cups water 1 1/2 cups canned chickpeas 1/2 cup fresh chopped parsley 1 tablespoon all purpose flour 2 garlic cloves, minced 2 tablespoons breadcrumbs 1 tablespoon olive oil Salt, pepper (to taste)

Directions: Bring 2 cups water to a boil. Add bulgur and cook until water has been absorbed, let cool. Create a paste with the chickpeas by placing in food processor and pulsing. Add the paste and remaining ingredient list to the bulgur and combine. Using wet hands, form the mixture into a burger shape. Add one tablespoon of olive oil to frying pan and heat over medium. Cook burgers on each side approximately 5 minutes, until golden brown.

Tomato Eggplant Spinach Salad

Preparation time: 30 minutes Serves: 4

Ingredients:

1 large eggplant, cut into 3/4 inch slices 5 oz spinach 1 tbsp sun-dried tomatoes, chopped 1 tbsp oregano, chopped 1 tbsp parsley, chopped 1 tbsp fresh mint, chopped 1 tbsp shallot, chopped For dressing: 1/4 cup olive oil 1/2 lemon juice 1/2 tsp smoked paprika 1 tsp Dijon mustard 1 tsp tahini 2 garlic cloves, minced Pepper Salt

Directions: Place sliced eggplants into the large bowl and sprinkle with salt and set aside for minutes. In a small bowl mix together all dressing ingredients. Set aside. Heat grill to medium-high heat. In a large bowl, add shallot, sun-dried tomatoes, herbs, and spinach. Rinse eggplant slices and pat dry with paper towel. Brush eggplant slices with olive oil and grill on medium high heat for 3-4 minutes on each side. Let cool the grilled eggplant slices then cut into quarters. Add eggplant to the salad bowl and pour dressing over salad. Toss well. Serve and enjoy.

Cauliflower Radish Salad

Preparation time: 15 minutes Serves: 4

Ingredients:

12 radishes, trimmed and chopped 1 tsp dried dill 1 tsp Dijon mustard 1 tbsp cider vinegar 1 tbsp olive oil 1 cup parsley, chopped ½ medium cauliflower head, trimmed and chopped ½ tsp black pepper ¼ tsp sea salt

Directions:

In a mixing bowl, combine together cauliflower, parsley, and radishes. In a small bowl, whisk together olive oil, dill, mustard, vinegar, pepper, and salt. Pour dressing over salad and toss well. Serve immediately and enjoy.

Citrus Salad

Preparation Time:10 minutes Cooking Time:0 minuteServings: 8

Ingredients:

3 tbsp. freshly squeezed lemon juice 5 tbsp. olive oil 2 tsp. Dijon mustard 2 tbsp. honey 1 tbsp. shallot, minced 1 tbsp. fresh thyme, chopped Salt and pepper to taste 4 cups mixed salad greens 2 cups radicchio leaves, shredded 3 oranges, sliced 1 grapefruit, sliced ¼ cup pomegranate seeds

Directions:

Combine lemon juice, oil, mustard, honey, shallot, thyme, salt and pepper in a glass jar with lid. Arrange the salad greens and radicchio leaves in a salad bowl. Top with the oranges and grapefruit slices. Sprinkle top with the pomegranate seeds. Serve with the dressing on the side.

Spinach Salad

Preparation Time: 10 minutes Cooking Time: 0 minutes
Servings: 4

Ingredients:

2 tbsp. olive oil Salt and pepper to taste 4 tsp. vinegar 8 cups baby spinach 1 cup raspberries ¼ cup goat cheese, crumbled ¼ cup hazelnuts, toasted and chopped

Directions:

Combine the vinegar, salt, pepper and oil in a bowl. Toss the spinach and raspberries in this mixture. Top with the goat cheese and hazelnuts. Lovely

Incredible Tomato Basil Soup

Servings: 6 Preparation time: 6 hours and 10 minutes

Ingredients:

1 cup of chopped celery 1 cup of chopped carrots 74 ounce of whole tomatoes, canned 2 cups of chopped white onion 2 teaspoons of minced garlic 1 tablespoon of salt 1/2 teaspoon of ground white pepper 1/4 cup of basil leaves and more for garnishing 1 bay leaf 32 fluid ounce of vegetable broth 1/2 cup of grated Parmesan cheese

Directions:

Using an 8 quarts or larger slow cooker, place all the ingredients. Stir until it mixes properly and cover the top. Plug in the slow cooker; adjust the cooking time to 5 hours and let it cook on the high heat setting or until the vegetables are tender. Blend the soup with a submersion blender or until soup reaches your desired state. Garnish it with the cheese, basil leaves and serve.

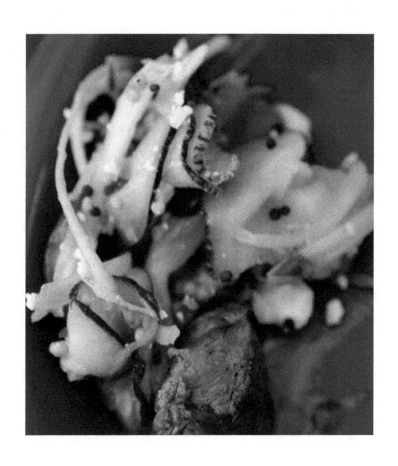

Spinach, Strawberry & Avocado Salad

Preparation Time: 5 minutes Cooking Time: 0 minute
Servings: 2

Ingredients:

6 cups baby spinach

1 cup strawberries, sliced

2 tbsp. onion, chopped

½ avocado, diced

4 tbsp. vinaigrette

4 tbsp. walnuts, toasted

Directions:

Toss the spinach, strawberries, onion and avocado in the
vinaigrette. Sprinkle with the walnuts.

Savory Squash & Apple Dish

Servings: 6 Preparation time: 4 hours and 15 minutes

Ingredients:

8 ounce of dried cranberries 4 medium-sized apples, peeled, cored and chopped 3 pounds of butternut squash, peeled, seeded and cubed Half of a medium-sized white onion, peeled and diced 1 tablespoon of ground cinnamon 1 1/2 teaspoons of ground nutmeg

Directions:

Take a 6-quarts slow cooker, grease it with a non-stick cooking spray and place the ingredients in it. Stir properly and cover the top. Plug in the slow cooker; adjust the cooking time to 4 hours and let it cook on the low heat setting or until it cooks thoroughly. Serve right away.

Wonderful Steamed Artichoke

Servings: 4 Preparation time: 4 hours and 5 minutes

Ingredients:

8 medium-sized artichokes, stemmed and trimmed 2 teaspoons of salt 4 tablespoons of lemon juice

Directions:

Cut 1-inch part of the artichoke from the top and place it in a 6-quarts slow cooker, facing an upright position. Using a bowl, place the lemon juice and pour in the salt until it mixes properly. Pour this mixture over the artichoke and add the water to cover at least ¾ of the artichokes. Cover the top, plug in the slow cooker; adjust the cooking time to 4 hours and let it cook on the high heat setting or until the artichokes get soft. Serve immediately.

Tangy Corn Chowder

Servings: 6 Preparation time: 5 hours and 15 minutes

Ingredients:

24 ounce of cooked kernel corn 3 medium-sized potatoes, pee led and diced 2 red chile peppers, minced 1 large white onion, peeled and diced 1 teaspoon of minced garlic 2 teaspoons of salt 1/2 teaspoon of ground black pepper 1 tablespoon of red chili powder 1 tablespoon of dried parsley 1/4 cup of vegan margarine 14 fluid ounce of soy milk 1 lime, juiced 24 fluid ounce of vegetable broth

Directions:

Using a 6-quarts slow cooker place all the ingredients except for the soy milk, margarine, and lime juice. Stir properly and cover it with the lid. Then plug in the slow cooker and let it cook for 3 to 4 hours at the high setting or until it is cooked thoroughly. When done, process the mixture with an immersion blender or until it gets smooth. Pour in the milk, margarine and stir properly. Continue cooking the soup for 1 hour at the low heat setting. Drizzle it with the lime juice and serve.

Eggplant Salad

Preparation Time: 15 minutes Cooking time: 25 minutes
Servings: 6

Ingredients:

2 eggplants 1 teaspoon salt 1 white onion, diced 1
teaspoon Pink salt 1 oz fresh cilantro 3 tablespoon lemon
juice 4 tablespoon olive oil 1 garlic clove, peeled

Directions:

Cut eggplants into halves. Preheat oven to 365F. Put
eggplants in the oven and cook for 25 minutes or until
they are tender. Meanwhile, blend diced onion and
transfer in the cheesecloth. Pour olive oil and lemon juice
in the bowl. Squeeze blended onion in the oil mixture.
Add salt. Chop cilantro and grind garlic. Add ingredients
in the oily mixture too. Stir it. Remove the eggplants from
the oven and chill them little. Remove the flesh from the
eggplants and transfer in the salad bowl. Add oil mixture
and stir gently.

"Potato" Salad

Preparation Time: 10 minutes Cooking time: 15 minutes
Servings: 4

Ingredients:

8 oz turnip, peeled 1 carrot, peeled 1 bay leaf ¼ teaspoon
peppercorns 1 teaspoon salt ½ teaspoon cayenne pepper
1 tablespoon fresh parsley, chopped 3 eggs, boiled 3
tablespoon sour cream 1 tablespoon mustard 2 cups
water, for vegetables

Directions:

Put turnip and carrot in the saucepan. Add water,
peppercorns, bay leaf, and salt. Close the lid and boil
vegetables for 15 minutes over high heat. The cooked
vegetables should be tender. Meanwhile, peel eggs and
chop them. Put the chopped eggs in the bowl. Sprinkle
them with cayenne pepper and chopped parsley. In the
separate bowl stir together mustard and sour cream.
When the vegetables are cooked, strain them and
transfer in the salad bowl. Add mustard sauce and stir.

Chunky Potato Soup

Servings: 6 Preparation time: 6 hours and 10 minutes

Ingredients:

1 medium-sized carrot, grated 6 medium-sized potatoes, peeled and diced 2 stalks of celery, diced 1 medium-sized white onion, peeled and diced 2 teaspoons of minced garlic 1 1/2 teaspoons of salt 1 teaspoon of ground black pepper 1 1/2 teaspoons of dried sage 1 teaspoon of dried thyme 2 tablespoons of olive oil 2 bay leaves 8 1/2 cups of vegetable water

Directions:

Using a 6-quarts slow cooker, place all the ingredients and stir properly. Cover it with the lid, plug in the slow cooker and let it cook for 6 hours at the high heat setting or until the potatoes are tender. Serve right away.

Simple Bechamel Sauce

Preparation Time: 30minutes Servings: 8

Ingredients:

3 tablespoons vegan butter 2 tablespoons flour 2 cups unheated milk Season the salt and pepper A pinch of nutmeg (optional)

Directions: Melt the butter in a saucepan over medium heat. Add the flour and beat until thick and bubbly but not browned (approximately 2 minutes). Pour the warm milk into the pan and continue stirring until the sauce has thickened (approximately 3 minutes). Add salt, pepper and nutmeg to the pan and stir. Use it immediately or, if done beforehand, put wax paper over the sauce until ready to use.

Spicy Cheese Sauce

Preparation Time: 10minutes

Ingredients:

1/2 teaspoon paprika 1/4 tsp Chipotle pepper powder 1/2 teaspoon sea salt (more to taste) 1 teaspoon Cumin (more to taste)

Directions:

Put all the INGREDIENTS in a powerful blender. Mix everything smooth and creamy. Adjust the spices to taste and add more water to obtain the desired consistency.

Homemade Worcestershire Sauce

Preparation Time: 30minutes

Ingredients:

1 cup apple cider vinegar 1/3 cup dark molasses 1/4 cup tamari 1/4 cup of water 3 tablespoons lemon juice 1 1/2 tablespoons salt 1/2 tablespoon dried mustard powder 1 teaspoon onion powder 3/4 teaspoon ground ginger 1/2 teaspoon black pepper 1/4 teaspoon garlic powder 1/4 teaspoon cayenne pepper 1/4 teaspoon ground cinnamon 1/8 teaspoon ground cloves or allspice 1/8 teaspoon ground cardamom

Directions:

Mix all the INGREDIENTS in a blender. Pour the mixture into a medium size saucepan and boil. Remove from heat and pour into a sterile beer glass or a clean 12.7 oz beer bottle or cider with a tight lid or lid. Store in the fridge. let it remain that way for a long time!

Tempeh Finger Fries

Preparation time: 10 minutes

Cooking time: 25 minutes Servings: 4.

Ingredients:

8 ounces fry-sliced tempeh 1 tbsp. olive oil 2 tbsp. soy sauce 1 tsp. chili powder

Directions:

Begin by heating up the soy sauce and the olive oil together in a skillet for about two minutes. Afterwards, add the sliced tempeh, making sure to coat the tempeh with the sauce. Add the chili powder and stir well. Sauté this mixture well for about seven or eight minutes. The tempeh should be crisp on all sides. Enjoy with your favorite dip!

Freedom Sweet Fries

Preparation time: 10 minutesCooking time: 45 minutes Servings: 4.

Ingredients:

2 sliced sweet potato fries 1 tsp. paprika 2 tsp. olive oil ½ tsp. cumin 1 tsp. salt

Directions:

Begin by preheating the oven to 350 degrees Fahrenheit. Next, stir together the sweet potatoes and all of the above ingredients in a large mixing bowl. Make sure to completely coat the sweet potato fries. Next, spread the sweet potato fries out on a baking sheet, and allow them to bake for fifty minutes. Serve warm, and enjoy

Cauliflower Steaks

Serves: 4 Preparation Time: 30 Minutes

Ingredients:

¼ Teaspoon Black Pepper ½ Teaspoon Sea Salt, Fine 1 Tablespoon Olive Oil 1 Head Cauliflower, Large ¼ Cup Creamy Hummus 2 Tablespoons Lemon Sauce ½ Cup Peanuts, Crushed (Optional)

Directions:

Start by heating your oven to 425. Cut your cauliflower stems, and then remove the leaves. Put the cut side down, and then slice half down the middle. Cut into ¾ inch steaks. If you cut them thinner, they could fall apart. Arrange them in a single layer on a baking sheet, drizzling with oil. Season and bake for twenty to twenty-five minutes. They should be lightly browned and tender. Spread your hummus on the steaks, drizzling with your lemon sauce. Top with peanuts if you're using it. Interesting Facts: Cauliflower: This vegetable is an extremely high source of vitamin A, vitamin B1, B2 and B3.

Tofu & Asparagus Stir Fry

Serves: 3 Time: 20 Minutes

Ingredients:

1 Tablespoon Ginger, Peeled & Grated

8 Ounces Firm Tofu, Chopped into Slices

4 Green Onions, Sliced Thin Toasted Sesame Oil to Taste

1 Bunch Asparagus, Trimmed & Chopped

1 Handful Cashew Nuts, Chopped & Toasted

2 Tablespoons Hoisin Sauce

1 Lime, Juiced & Zested

1 Handful Mint, Fresh & Chopped

1 Handful Basil, Fresh & Chopped

3 Cloves Garlic, Chopped

3 Handfuls Spinach, Chopped Pinch Sea Salt

Directions:

Get out a wok and heat up your oil. Add in your tofu, cooking for a few minutes. Put your tofu to the side, and then sauté your red pepper flakes, ginger, salt, onions and asparagus for a minute. Mix in your spinach, garlic, and cashews, cooking for another two minutes. Add your tofu back in, and then drizzle in your lime juice, lime zest, hoisin sauce, cooking for another half a minute. Remove it from heat, adding in your mint and basil. Interesting Facts: Sesame seeds can be easily added to crackers, bread, salads, and stir-fry meals. Bonus: Help in lowering cholesterol and high blood pressure. Double bonus: Help with asthma, arthritis, and migraines!

Cream of Mushroom Soup

Preparation time: 5 minutes Cooking time: 12 minutes
Servings: 6

Ingredients:

1 medium white onion, peeled, chopped 16 ounces button mushrooms, sliced 1 ½ teaspoon minced garlic 1/4 cup all-purpose flour 1/2 teaspoon ground black pepper 1 teaspoon dried thyme 1/4 teaspoon nutmeg 1/2 teaspoon salt 2 tablespoons vegan butter 4 cups vegetable broth 1 1/2 cups coconut milk, unsweetened

Directions:

Take a large pot, place it over medium-high heat, add butter and when it melts, add onions and garlic, stir in garlic and cook for 5 minutes until softened and nicely brown. Then sprinkle flour over vegetables, continue cooking for 1 minute, then add remaining ingredients, stir until mixed and simmer for 5 minutes until thickened. Serve straight away

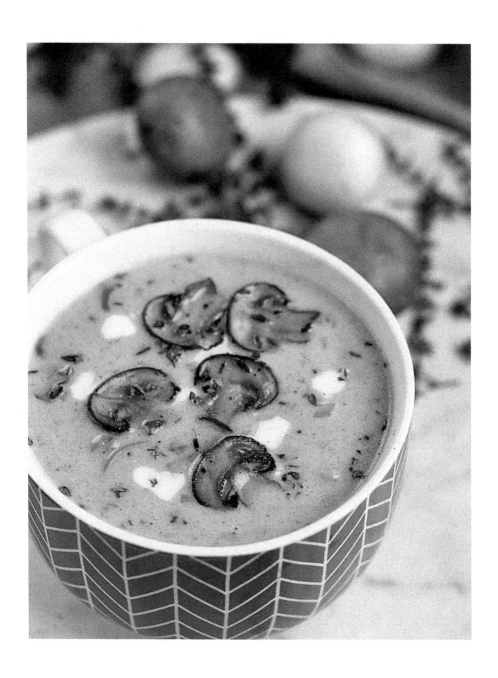

Lentil Soup

Preparation time: 5 minutes Cooking time: 40 minutes
Servings: 6

Ingredients:

1 cup brown lentils 1 medium white onion, peeled,
chopped 28 ounces diced tomatoes 1 ½ teaspoon minced
garlic 1 inch of ginger, grated 3 cups vegetable broth 1/2
teaspoon salt 2 tablespoons curry powder 1 teaspoon
cumin 1/2 teaspoon cayenne 1 tablespoon olive oil 1 1/2
cups coconut milk, unsweetened ¼ cup chopped cilantro

Directions:

Take a soup pot, place it over medium-high heat, add oil
and when hot, add onion, stir in garlic and ginger and
cook for 5 minutes until golden brown. Then add all the
ingredients except for milk and cilantro, stir until mixed
and simmer for 25 minutes until lentils have cooked.
When done, stir in milk, cook for 5 minutes until
thoroughly heated and then garnish the soup with
cilantro. Serve straight away

Mexican Lentil Soup

Preparation time: 5 minutes Cooking time: 45 minutes

Servings: 6

Ingredients:

2 cups green lentils

1 medium red bell pepper, cored, diced

1 medium white onion, peeled, diced

2 cups diced tomatoes

8 ounces diced green chilies

2 celery stalks, diced

2 medium carrots, peeled, diced

1 ½ teaspoon minced garlic

1/2 teaspoon salt

1 tablespoon cumin

1/4 teaspoon smoked paprika

1 teaspoon oregano

1/8 teaspoon hot sauce

2 tablespoons olive oil

8 cups vegetable broth

¼ cup cilantro, for garnish

1 avocado, peeled, pitted, diced, for garnish

Directions:

Take a large pot over medium heat, add oil and when hot, add all the vegetables, reserving tomatoes and chilies, and cook for 5 minutes until softened. Then add garlic, stir in oregano, cumin, and paprika, and continue cooking for 1 minute. Add lentils, tomatoes and green chilies, season with salt, pour in the broth and simmer the soup for 40 minutes until cooked. When done, ladle soup into bowls, top with avocado and cilantro and serve straight away

Cauliflower Soup

Preparation time: 10 minutes Cooking time: 40 minutes
Servings: 2

Ingredients:

1 small head of cauliflower, cut into florets 4 tablespoons
pomegranate seeds 2 sprigs of thyme and more for
garnishing 1 teaspoon minced garlic 2/3 teaspoon salt
1/3 teaspoon ground black pepper 1 tablespoon olive oil
1 1/2 cups vegetable stock 1/2 cup coconut milk,
unsweetened

Directions:

Take a pot, place it over medium heat, add oil and when
hot, add garlic and cook for 1 minute until fragrant. Add
florets, thyme, pour in the stock and bring the mixture
to boil. Switch heat to the medium low level, simmer the
soup for 30 minutes until florets are tender, then remove
the pot from heat, discard the thyme and puree using an
immersion blender until smooth. Stir milk into the soup,
season with salt and black pepper, then garnish with
pomegranate seeds and thyme sprigs and serve.

Asparagus Soup

Preparation time: 10 minutes Cooking time: 20 minutes Servings: 4

Ingredients:

1/2 head of medium cauliflower, cut into florets 1 medium white onion, peeled, sliced 2 pounds asparagus, ends trimmed, chopped 2 teaspoons minced garlic ½ teaspoon ground black pepper 1/2 cup nutritional yeast ½ teaspoon salt 1 lemon, juiced 1 tablespoon olive oil 6 cups vegetable broth

Directions:

Take a large stockpot, place it over medium-high heat, add oil and when hot, add onions and garlic, and cook for 7 minutes until onions are translucent. Then add cauliflower florets and asparagus, pour in vegetable broth, bring to boil, then switch heat to medium level and simmer for 10 minutes until vegetables are tender. Puree soup by using an immersion blender, then return it over medium heat, season with salt and black pepper, stir in lemon juice and yeast and serve straight away.

Butternut Squash and Coconut Milk

Soup Preparation time: 10 minutes Cooking time: 35 minutes Servings: 6

Ingredients:

1 cup diced parsnips 2 cups diced sweet potato 1 large sweet onion, peeled, diced 1 ½ cups diced carrots 4 cups diced butternut squash 2 teaspoons minced garlic 1/4 teaspoon ground ginger ¼ teaspoon ground black pepper ½ teaspoon of sea salt 1/4 teaspoon ground allspice 1 teaspoon poultry seasoning 1 teaspoon pumpkin pie spice 1/4 teaspoon ground cinnamon 32 ounces vegetable stock 14 ounces coconut milk, unsweetened

Directions:

Take a large Dutch oven, place it over medium heat, add onions, drizzle with 2 tablespoons water and cook for 5 minutes until softened, drizzling with more 2 tablespoons at a time if required. Then stir in garlic, cook for another minute, switch heat to the high level, add remaining ingredients, reserving milk, salt, and black pepper, and bring the soup to boil. Then switch heat to medium-low level and simmer for 20 minutes until vegetables are tender. When done, puree soup by using an immersion blender, then stir in coconut milk, season with salt and black pepper and cook for 3 minutes until warm. Serve straight away

Potato and Kale Soup

Preparation time: 5 minutes Cooking time: 15 minutes Servings: 2

Ingredients:

1 small white onion, peeled, chopped 2 ½ cups cubed potatoes 2 cups leek, cut into rings 1/2 cup chopped carrots 1/2 cup chopped celery ½ teaspoon minced garlic 2/3 teaspoon salt 1/3 teaspoon ground black pepper 1 tablespoon olive oil 3 1/2 cups vegetable broth 1 cup kale, cut into stripes Croutons, for serving

Directions:

Take a large pot, place it over medium heat, add oil and when hot, add onion and cook for 2 minutes until sauté. Stir in garlic, cook for another minute, then add all the vegetables and continue cooking for 3 minutes. Pour in broth, cook for 15 minutes, then add kale and cook for 2 minutes until tender. Season soup with salt and black pepper, puree by using an immersion blender until smooth, then top with croutons and serve.

Roasted Cauliflower Soup

Preparation time: 10 minutes Cooking time: 60 minutes Servings: 4

Ingredients:

1 medium head of cauliflower, cut into florets 1 small white onion, peeled, diced 1 medium carrot, peeled, diced 1 stalk of celery, diced 1 head of garlic, top off 2/3 teaspoon salt 1/3 teaspoon ground black pepper 1 teaspoon smoked paprika 2 tablespoons nutritional yeast 1 teaspoon hot smoked paprika 4 tablespoons olive oil 12 ounces coconut milk, unsweetened 4 cups vegetable broth ½ cup chopped parsley

Directions: Switch on the oven, then set it to 400 degrees F and let it preheat. Place top off garlic on a piece of foil, drizzle with 1 tablespoon oil, and then wrap. Place cauliflower florets in a bowl, drizzle with 2 tablespoons oil, season with salt and black pepper, and toss until well coated. Take a baking sheet, spread cauliflower florets in it in a single layer, add wrapped garlic and bake for 30 minutes until roasted. Then place a large pot over medium-high heat, add remaining oil and when hot, add onions and cook for 3 minutes. Then add celery and carrot, continue cooking for 3 minutes, season with salt and paprika, pour in broth, and bring it to a boil. Add roasted garlic and florets, bring the mixture to boil, then switch heat to medium-low level and simmer for 15 minutes. Puree the soup by using an immersion blender, stir in milk and yeast until mixed and simmer for 3 minutes until hot. Garnish soup with parsley and then serve.

Ramen Noodle Soup

Preparation time: 10 minutes Cooking time: 20 minutes
Servings: 2

Ingredients:

For The Mushrooms and Tofu: 2 cups sliced shiitake
mushrooms 6 ounces tofu, extra-firm, drained, sliced 1
tablespoon olive oil 1 tablespoon soy sauce

For the Noodle Soup: 2 packs of dried ramen noodles
1 medium carrot, peeled, grated 1 inch of ginger, grated
1 teaspoon minced garlic ¾ cup baby spinach leaves 1
tablespoon olive oil 6 cups vegetable broth

For Garnish: Sesame seeds as needed Soy sauce as
needed Sriracha sauce as needed

Directions: Prepare mushrooms and tofu and for this,
place tofu pieces in a plastic bag, add soy sauce, seal the
bag and turn it upside until tofu is coated. Take a skillet
pan, place it over medium heat, add oil and when hot,
add tofu slices and cook for 5 to 10 minutes until crispy
and browned on all sides, flipping frequently and when
done, set aside until required. Add mushrooms into the
pan, cook for 8 minutes until golden, pour soy sauce from

tofu pieces in it, and stir until coated. Meanwhile, prepare noodle soup and for this, take a soup pot, place it over medium-high heat, add oil and when hot, add garlic and ginger and cook for 1 minute until fragrant. Then pour in the broth, bring the mixture to boil, add noodles and cook until tender. Then stir spinach into the noodle soup, remove the pot from heat and distribute evenly between bowls. Add mushrooms and tofu along with garnishing and then serve.

Hot and Sour Soup

Preparation time: 5 minutes Cooking time: 20 minutes Servings: 4

Ingredients: 2 tablespoons dried wood ears 3.5 ounces bamboo shoots, sliced into thin strips 1 medium carrot, peeled, sliced into thin strips 5 dried shiitake mushrooms 1 tablespoon grated ginger 1 teaspoon minced garlic 1 teaspoon ground black pepper 1 teaspoon salt 1/4 cup soy sauce 1 teaspoon sugar 1/2 cup rice vinegar 4 cups vegetable stock 1 1/2 cup water, boiling 7.5 ounces tofu, extra-firm, drained 1 tablespoon green onion tops, chopped ¼ cup water, at room temperature 2 tablespoons cornstarch 1 teaspoon sesame oil

Directions: Take a small bowl, place wood ears in it, then pour in boiling water until covered and let stand for 30 minutes. Meanwhile, take another bowl, place mushrooms in it, pour in 1 ½ cup water and let the mushrooms stand for 30 minutes. After 30 minutes, drain the wood ears, rinse well and cut into slices, remove and discard the hard bits. Similarly, drain the mushrooms, reserving their soaking liquid and slice the mushrooms, removing and discarding their stems. Take a large pot, place it over medium-high heat, add all the ingredients including reserved mushroom liquid, leave the last five ingredients, stir well and bring the mixture to boil. Then switch heat to medium level and simmer the soup for 10 minutes until cooked. Meanwhile, place cornstarch in a bowl, add water at room temperature, and stir well until smooth. Cut tofu into 1-inch pieces, add into the simmering soup along with cornstarch mixture, and continue to simmer the soup until it reaches to desired thickness. Drizzle with sesame oil, distribute soup into bowls, garnish with green onions and serve.

Thai Coconut Soup

Preparation time: 10 minutes Cooking time: 15 minutes
Servings: 12

Ingredients:

2 mangos, peeled, cut into bite-size pieces 1/2 cup green lentils, cooked 2 sweet potatoes, peeled, cubed 1/2 cup quinoa, cooked 1 green bell pepper, cored, cut into strips ½ teaspoon chopped basil ½ teaspoon chopped rosemary 2 tablespoons red curry paste 1/4 cup mixed nut 2 teaspoons orange zest 30 ounces coconut milk, unsweetened

Directions:

Take a large saucepan, place it over medium-high heat, add sweet potatoes, pour in the milk and bring the mixture to boil. Then switch heat to medium-low level, add remaining ingredients, except for quinoa and lentils, stir and cook for 15 minutes until vegetables have softened. Then stir in quinoa and lentils, cook for 3 minutes until hot, and then serve.

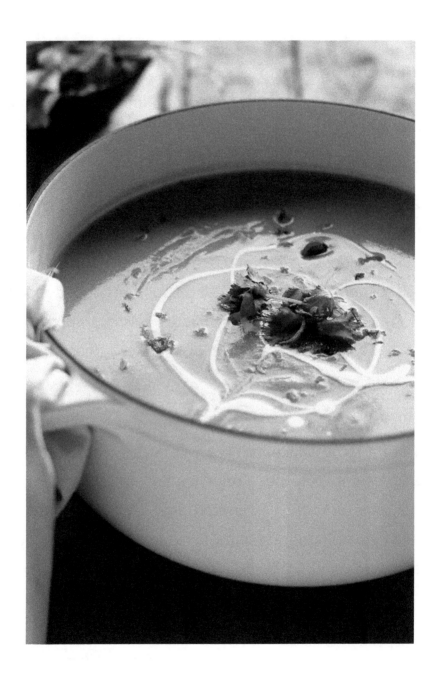

Pomegranate and Walnut Stew

Preparation time: 10 minutes Cooking time: 55 minutes

Servings: 6

Ingredients:

1 head of cauliflower, cut into florets 1 medium white onion, peeled, diced 1 1/2 cups California walnuts, toasted 1 cup yellow split peas 1 1/2 tablespoons honey ¼ teaspoon salt ½ teaspoon turmeric ½ teaspoon cinnamon 2 tablespoons olive oil, separated 4 cups pomegranate juice 2 tablespoons chopped parsley 2 tablespoons chopped walnuts, for garnishing

Directions:

Take a medium saute pan, place it over medium heat, add walnuts, cook for 5 minutes until toasted and then cool for 5 minutes. Transfer walnuts to the food processor, pulse for 2 minutes until ground, and set aside until required. Take a large saute pan, place it over medium heat, add 1 tablespoon oil and when hot, add onion and cook for 5 minutes until softened. Switch heat to medium-low heat, then add lentils and walnuts, stir in cinnamon, salt, and turmeric, pour in honey and pomegranate, stir until mixed and simmer the mixture for 40 minutes until the sauce has reduced by half and lentils have softened. Meanwhile, place cauliflower florets in a food processor and then pulse for 2 minutes until mixture resembles rice. Take a medium to saute pan, place it over medium heat, add remaining oil and when hot, add cauliflower rice, cook for 5 minutes until softened, and then season with salt. Serve cooked pomegranate and walnut sauce with cooked cauliflower rice and garnish with walnuts and parsley.

Vegetarian Irish Stew

Preparation time: 5 minutes Cooking time: 38 minutes
Servings: 6

Ingredients:

1 cup textured vegetable protein, chunks ½ cup split red lentils 2 medium onions, peeled, sliced 1 cup sliced parsnip 2 cups sliced mushrooms 1 cup diced celery, 1/4 cup flour 4 cups vegetable stock 1 cup rutabaga 1 bay leaf ½ cup fresh parsley 1 teaspoon sugar ¼ teaspoon ground black pepper 1/4 cup soy sauce ¼ teaspoon thyme 2 teaspoons marmite ¼ teaspoon rosemary 2/3 teaspoon salt ¼ teaspoon marjoram

Directions:

Take a large soup pot, place it over medium heat, add oil and when it gets hot, add onions and cook for 5 minutes until softened. Then switch heat to the low level, sprinkle with flour, stir well, add remaining ingredients, stir until combined and simmer for 30 minutes until vegetables have cooked. When done, season the stew with salt and black pepper and then serve.

Spinach and Cannellini Bean Stew

Preparation time: 10 minutes Cooking time: 15 minutes
Servings: 6

Ingredients:

28 ounces cooked cannellini beans

24 ounces tomato passata

17 ounces spinach chopped

¼ teaspoon ground black pepper

2/3 teaspoon salt

1 ¼ teaspoon curry powder

1 cup cashew butter

¼ teaspoon cardamom

2 tablespoons olive oil

1 teaspoon salt

¼ cup cashews

2 tablespoons chopped basil

2 tablespoons chopped parsley

Directions:

Take a large saucepan, place it over medium heat, add 1 tablespoon oil and when hot, add spinach and cook for 3 minutes until fried. Then stir in butter and tomato passata until well mixed, bring the mixture to a near boil, add beans and season with ¼ teaspoon curry powder, black pepper, and salt. Take a small saucepan, place it over medium heat, add remaining oil, stir in cashew, stir in salt and curry powder and cook for 4 minutes until roasted, set aside until required. Transfer cooked stew into a bowl, top with roasted cashews, basil, and parsley, and then serve.

Lightning Source UK Ltd.
Milton Keynes UK
UKHW020738270522
403610UK00001B/8